The Super Hero Structure

Daniel K. Arnold

Books By Daniel Arnold:

The Super Hero Manual

Ever-Changing

Black Bird

Obey God.

Journalists For Jesus

Guest Speakers In Mental Health

To Be A Man

#Satisfied

The Super Hero Structure- Chapter 1

Balance: Noun

3)Mental steadiness or emotional stability; habit of calm behavior, judgement, etc.

Dictionary.com

Sensitive: Adjective

3)Having acute mental or emotional sensibility; aware of and responsive to the feelings of others

Dictionary.com

Special effort must be taken by the diverse Super Hero to live a balanced life. Substance abuse, sleep deprivation, or any out of proportion activity can throw him/her off.

There is a time when too much effort can be exerted—workaholic. There is a time when too little effort can be exerted—idleness.

"With God all things are possible (Matthew 19:26)"—including stability.

Stable2: Adjective

1)Not likely to fall or give way as a structure support, foundation, etc.; firm, steady

Dictionary.com

How can we live an abundant life that is also able to withstand the test of time?

How do we find balance as sensitive heroic beings?

I cashed in my chips. I was "cruising for a bruising." I finally found a cause worth obsessing over.

After over 100 successful days of not taking psychotropic drugs, I became passionate about the issue of child sex trafficking locally.

I cared not for sleep or mental stability. I gave night and day energy to the cause.

I quickly crashed.

"Man looks on the outward appearance, but God looks on the heart (1 Samuel 16:7)."

I appeared to be a fool to many people in the choices I made in living every moment as if it were my last.

I was told I needed self-care. My response was what about those children locked in basements with duct tape over their mouths. Their screams were silenced and I wanted to be their voice!

I stepped out of balance. I stepped out of the norm. I do not regret it.

Albeit, I was not perfect, but only human. I would compare myself to the zeal of the disciple Peter who chopped off a servant's ear when Jesus was arrested.

I simply wanted to make a dent in the issue. (I still do.) I wanted people to respond outrageously with me because exploited children matter!

My obsession landed me back in a mental hospital and ending my favorite job.

Oh well. No regrets.

Super heroes live it large making large mistakes and large advancements. At the end of the day, we are accountable to God.

Thank you Jesus that someone is hearing me out. Give your all to Jesus whatever it costs.

We can never out give what Jesus gave for us!

What would it look like if we ran after following God with reckless abandomment—no fear growing closer and closer.

"Our Father who art in Heaven. Holy is thy name. Thy Kingdom come. Thy will be done on earth as it is in Heaven. Give us this day our daily bread and forgive us our sins as we forgive those who sin against us. Lead us not into temptation but deliver us from evil. For thine is the Kingdom and the glory forever and ever (Matthew 6:9-13)."

Help us with that which we do not understand.

God gives His radical Super Heroes an abundant life—like Heaven.

Abundant: Adjective
1. Present in great quantity; more than adequate; oversufficient

Dictionary.com

"Let your soul delight in fatness (Isaiah 55:2)."

God wants us to walk a special journey with Him that is meaningful and overflowing with blessing—like a waterfall.

Wooo….. Just want to share it!

As I move past this season that seems radical to others, spending a great deal of time in the hospital, I move forward towards the structured Super Hero life.

I do not regret my past, nor my present. I continue to make mistakes, but I am not here to please people.

"But the Comforter, which is the Holy Ghost, whom the Father with send in my name, He will teach you all things and bring all things to your remembrance, whatsoever I have spoken unto you (Jesus, John 14:26)."

I commune with the Living God! He comforts me. He brings me balance.

The Super Hero Struture – Chapter 2

One of the hardest parts of my life was, for whatever reason, over year ago, I felt lead by the Lord to resist psychotropic medications.

I was inside a mental hospital receiving daily shots of Haldol to my hip. Few can understand why I chose to endure this daily torture, but I was seeking to follow God to the best of my ability.

Remember, every super hero is a unique servant of the Lord on a unique journey. There is a right and wrong, but morals can be complex.

One man eats meat. Another man eats only vegetables. Do not judge another servant of the Lord.

This resistance built in me the backbone I have today. Yes, eventually I found myself taking medications orally, but this experience I carry in my heart as I decided to follow God no matter what.

The Super Hero Structure – Chapter 3

Today, I have found medication that allow me to function normally. I drink coffee in the morning to pick me up.

Life is abundant, but difficult adventures continue every day.

Daily is a new chapter. I have been arrested for putting Bibles in front of me to pass out at Justice in Mental Health Organization Drop-In Center.

I have been relocated from the sidewalk for obstructing it. All this has pointed me to my calling:

Literary Free Zone

Yes! The Lord knows what is best. He has helped me to develop "The Super Hero Structure."

The Super Hero Structure – Chapter 4 – The Daily Grind

Everyone needs a schedule. Everyone needs structure. Everyone needs to be a productive member of society.

Unfortunately, Super Heroes have seemed to have burned many epic bridges going full tilt!

Praise the Lord! God has a plan for us. Perhaps we receive disability money and have serious setbacks to work.

There are agencies that can help with this. If it is still hard to work, perhaps entrepreneurship is in order.

The Literary Free Zone has been created as a positive opportunity to develop a daily structured schedule.

All I do is simply pass out literature, talk and pray with people in the park on a consistent basis.

I commit up to 40 hours a week to this project—approximately 8am-4pm, Monday through Friday.

I receive donations from many compassionate individuals who want to help the poor with spiritual literature and food.

This structure along with a big breakfast (coffee included) give me something to wake up to in the morning.

After I was sent away from JIMHO where I initiated the Literary Free Zone, I was initially depressed. I felt like I wanted to stop living, but God had a plan.

After being removed from the sidewalk by a police officer, I found a park that welcomes all.

I love these people, children of God. They can come and spend time with me. We can reach out and develop a positive environment. This is my forty hour work week.

The Super Hero Structure –

Chapter 5 – Sabbath

An element of finding balance as a Super Hero is finding a lull period. There must be downtime. We need to keep the Sabbath holy.

I take my Sabbath days typically at Advent House. This beautiful place meets food needs as well as sharing some wonderful sermons.

They need financial help. Please call: 517-485-4722

The Super Hero Structure –

Chapter 6 – Rest

Now that everything has slowed down, battles have been found fought, I want to live a long fruitful life.

God promises us sweet sleep. Without meds, I sleep a lot less. It seems that the right med combo works for me now.

I have been on many different prescriptions. I believe in never giving up and self-advocating for what is needed until I find the right balance.

Serve the Lord. Go to bed at routine night times.

I take care of myself and pamper myself when I feel exhausted.

I continue my 40 hour schedule as much as possible for the sake of routine and getting in the positive groove.

The Super Hero Structure –

Chapter 7

We matter. We must not ever give up. We must find a reason to be grateful for all seasons of life.

God is good and He loves us. He has compassion on the broken. God wants to use us to make a difference in the lives of others.

We have a purpose and past struggles become a part of our story to help the needy.

The Super Hero Structure – Chapter 8 – Accountability

As much as I enjoy going on my own journey, there is danger in exploring life as a "lone wolf."

We need accountability with solid Christians who have experienced some tangles in life.

Thank you Jesus that "iron sharpens iron," as "one man sharpens another (Proverbs 27:17)."

We have a lot we can learn from other perspectives. I recommend the counsel of multiple people.

The Super Hero Structure – Chapter 9 – What's Next

"Do not worry about tomorrow, for tomorrow will take care of itself. There are enough worries in today (Matthew 6:34)."

God has our back. Let's keep serving Him and stop worrying. Let's climb into the Word of God and talk with Him.

He walks with me, talks with me, and comforts me. I know my future is blessed as long as I continue in His kindness.

Trials may come, but also peace. We need to be faithful with what is put before us. God brings the increase!

I have lived a passionate life and now I just want to live the life God has for me. Through patient affliction, I will not rush the will of God, but I will wait on God's direction whatever the cost!

Lord, prepare me if suffering is in my future. Give me the strength to always be on watch to be found serving Jesus when He returns.

The threat of torture puts fear in me a little, but the Bible says we will "not be tempted beyond what we can bear (1 Corinthians 10:13)."

Oh Lord, prepare me for whatever is ahead.

The Super Hero Structure – Chapter 10

We can make a difference, change, impact. Relax and realize "All things are possible with God (Matthew 19:26)."

"Unless the Lord builds the house the laborers build in vain (Psalm 127:1)."

"Forgetting what is behind and pressing on to what is ahead, I run as to get the prize of the high calling of Jesus Christ (Philippians 3:13)."

The Super Hero Structure – Chapter 11

Every super hero has an innate desire to make a difference in society. Sometimes we feel alone and want to socialize at odd hours.

It is difficult to turn off the stimulation/excitement many times.

The Bible says in Psalm 23, "He maketh me to lie down in green pastures."

Thank you God for allowing me to be humbled at the right times. Thank you for putting me in the right places at the right times. It is truly a blessing in disguise.

The Super Hero Structure – Chapter 12

An important element to the Super Hero Structure is tuning into the Voice of God. The Great Comforter has our best interest at heart.

For clarity, we must follow the commands of the Bible to confess Jesus as Lord, believe He was raised from the dead, and be baptized in the name of Jesus with a repentant heart.

"Repent and be baptized in the name of Jesus, for the remission of sins, and the Holy Ghost shall come upon you (Acts 2:38)."

"Be still and know that I am God. I will be exalted above the nations (Psalm 46:10)."

Jesus has our best interest at heart. Be still before Him.

Many times we seek out a feel good life when God wants us to slow down and ask Him for help.

"Do not be anxious about anything, but in everything, with prayer and petition, with thanksgiving, present your requests to God. And the peace of God which surpasses all understanding will guard your hearts and mind in Christ Jesus (Philippians 4:6-7)."

With the peace of God, we hear His still small voice.

When we do not know what to pray, Jesus told how we ought to pray.

"Our Father,
Who art in Heaven,

Holy is your name,

Your Kingdom come,

Your will be done,

On Earth as it is in Heaven.

Give us our daily bread,

And forgiveth our sins,

As we forgive those who sin against us,

And deliver us from evil,

For yours is the Kingdom and the Glory forever and ever. Amen (Matthew 6:9-13)."

"The effectual, fervent prayer of a righteous man availeth much (James 5:16)."

If there is something between you and God, confess it. Experience restoration!

"If we confess our sins, He is faithful and just to forgive our sins and to cleanse us from all unrighteousness (1 John 1:9)."

Be still before God. Put your plea before God on paper. Document answered prayer.

Always give thanks through the whole process.

Be satisfied!

Write to God and let God write back to you with that still, small voice.

Hallelujah!

If everything seems to go wrong, slow down, give thanks and ask God for help. He is faithful.

The Super Hero Structure – Chapter 13 – The Daily Grind

One of my quirks is that I dread doing regular exercise or physical labor.

Turns out I am compelled to pull my wagon one mile each direction to and from my park ministry site. I move all my materials up and down the stairs.

The Lord frequently leads me where I do not feel like going for my benefit. This routine exercise is part of my Super Hero Structure. Thank you Jesus!

The Super Hero Structure –

Chapter 14 – Cheats

Some people on diets say it is good to cheat once in awhile and enjoy a treat.

It is helpful for the Super Hero not be too rigid. Occasionally, he/she might stay up with not enough sleep. Occasionally, he/she might consume treats or enjoy laid back recreational activities, even planning to divert from schedule.

The importance is moderation, following the lead of God and always to be thankful.

"His praise shall continually be on my lips (Psalm 34:1)."

The Super Hero Structure –

Chapter 15 – When It Rains

Life is not always ideal from the Super Hero vantage point. Disasters come heavy, but the sun does come out.

Come out of seclusion Mighty Warrior! Stop hiding and enjoy the seasons of change that build us.

Before we know it, the weather changes. Experience the life God has made for us now!

Get up and be active! Take a walk. Go to church. Eat at a cook-out. Try a little labor to help others.

We will be surprised at what God makes possible if we give Him a chance. When we wait on the Lord, we need not be shocked when the sun comes out to shine.

The Super Hero Structure – Chapter 16 – Results

We have to ask ourselves if results are measured by mass popular response or actual discipleship impact.

Sometimes the diverse Super Hero can feel alone in his/her efforts. He/she must remember that Jesus our Savior, who changed and changes the world experienced desert moments Himself.

Popular response does not reflect reality.

We must press on. Jesus prayed in the Garden before He was betrayed. His own disciples failed to stand watch with Him.

They went to sleep when Jesus asked them to pray. Oh God, may we not let you down in this way. In quiet moments, may we fellowship with you.

May we talk with the Holy Ghost. May we never give up as Super Heroes!

God is doing something special in us that is unseen. We are like baby trees developing roots as we struggle to push through. It doesn't matter if people are Nay-Sayers.

We push on!

The Super Hero Structure – Chapter 17 – Faith

Do we believe God has allowed us to be in our current season for a reason? Do we believe that "with God all things are possible (Matthew 19:26)?"

This is our hour and season. Opportunity knows no matter what the world says.

We have hope and a future. God rewards those who diligently seek Him.

Consider God's servant, David, son of Jesse. He was mostly invisible, but God chose him to rule as King of Israel!

He was God's beloved. We can be the same. We are called as

Super Heroes. Life may seem messy and wasted, but God is a redeemer of the time. Let us put our full trust in Him.

"…Perfect love casts out fear because fear has to do with torment. The man who fears is not made perfect in love (1 John 4:18)."

Follow God's way 100% no matter what the world says. Watch God expand our territory.

The Super Hero Structure – Chapter 18

Make a timestamp. Plan a memory. Jesus answers prayer. Write down the time, location, and date. Press your plea with thanksgiving and expect a great response.

Jesus answers prayer.

Write down the response you get. God is in the business of doing miracles for people of faith. Do not hesitate to ask. Nothing is too hard for God.

The Super Hero Structure – Chapter 19 – Privacy

God wants us to have special moments with just us and Him.

This can be expressed creatively through writing, a song, dancing, a prayer closet.

God has a wonderful plan for us that He wants to share with us.

He wants us to stop and quietly listen.

Hallelujah!

Have a private time with God.

The Super Hero Structure – Chapter 20 – Never Give Up

The Lord has a strong calling on our lives. We cannot give up. We need to reach out with thanksgiving.

We matter. We should seek help until we get it.

"…God is light and in Him is no darkness at all (1 John 1:5)."

Make wise choices. Gather in prayer with the brothers and sisters.

God cares about us!

"For God so loved the world that He gave His only Son that whosoever believeth in Him shall not perish but have everlasting life (John 3:16)."

The Super Hero Structure
Chapter 21

There is no conclusion to the abundant Christ-led life for the Super Hero!

We take it slow and live faithfully.

"You will keep him in perfect peace whose mind is stayed on you, because he trusts in you (Isaiah 26:3)."

Perfect peace is not worrying about anything; sharing everything with God. The Comforter, the Holy Spirit, is very real. Commune with Him all the time!

The blessing is upon us and we can forget yesterday's sorrows.

Live the blessed life of the Super Hero Structure, praising our Savior forever.

There is no rush, no panic to eternal paradise, "on earth as it is in Heaven (Matthew 6:10)."